COPING WITH A MODERN PLAGUE

Candida albicans is an insidious yeast infection that is growing in epidemic proportions. It affects mainly women in their childbearing years, but can strike anyone—even infants. It assumes a wide variety of symptomatic forms and can cause untold distress. But Candida victims can fight back—using a combination of diet, supplements and drugs to help wipe out this pest. And those who have been fortunate enough to escape Candida can upgrade their nutrition to optimal levels and thus strengthen their immune systems to help ward off the disease. This Good Health Guide sums it all up for you—diagnosis, treatment, prevention.

ABOUT THE AUTHOR AND EDITORS

Ray C. Wunderlich, Jr., received his M.D. degree from Columbia University. He is a board-certified pediatrician who now practices preventive medicine in St. Petersburg, Florida, where he is on the staff of two hospitals. He is an avid long-distance runner and the author of *Kids, Brains and Learning; Allergy, Brains and Children Coping; Improving Your Diet; Fatigue;* and *Sugar and Your Health*. Dr. Wunderlich is also coauthor, with Dwight Kalita, of *Nourishing Your Child*, published in 1984 by Keats Publishing.

Dwight K. Kalita received his doctorate from Bowling Green State University, where he was Assistant Professor and behavioral counselor. He is Research Director of the Bio-Ecologic Research Center in Defiance, Ohio, a non-profit, all-volunteer organization. He is also President of Midwest Microcomputers and a member of the Board of Directors of the Institute of Bio-Ecologic Medicine in St. Petersburg, Florida. He coauthored *Victory Over Diabetes* and *Brain Allergies: The Psychonutrient Connection* with William H. Philpott, M.D., and coedited *A Physician's Handbook on Orthomolecular Medicine* with Roger J. Williams, Ph.D. He writes frequently for a variety of general and professional publications.

Richard A. Passwater, Ph.D., is one of the most called-upon authorities for information relating to preventive health care. A noted biochemist, he is credited with popularizing the term "supernutrition" largely as a result of having written two bestsellers on the subject—*Supernutrition: Megavitamin Revolution* and *Supernutrition for Healthy Hearts*. His other books include *Easy No-Flab Diet, Cancer and Its Nutritional Therapies* and *Selenium as Food & Medicine*. His most recent books are *Trace Elements, Hair Analysis and Nutrition*, with Elmer M. Cranton, M.D., and the Good Health Guide *Beta-Carotene*.

Earl Mindell, R.Ph., Ph.D., combines the expertise and working experience of a pharmacist with extensive knowledge in most of the nutrition areas. His book *Earl Mindell's Vitamin Bible* is now a million-copy bestseller; and his more recent *Vitamin Bible for Your Kids* may very well duplicate his first *Bible*'s publishing history. Dr. Mindell's popular *Quick & Easy Guide to Better Health* was published by Keats Publishing.

CANDIDA ALBICANS
HOW TO FIGHT AN EXPLODING EPIDEMIC OF YEAST-RELATED DISEASES

by Ray C. Wunderlich, Jr., M.D., and
Dwight K. Kalita, Ph.D.

Keats Publishing, Inc.   New Canaan, Connecticut

Candida Albicans is not intended as medical advice. Its intention is solely informational and educational. Please consult a medical or health professional should the need for one be warranted.

Good Health Guides are published by Keats Publishing, Inc.
27 Pine Street (Box 876)
New Canaan, Connecticut 06840

Contents

INTRODUCTION

Each one of us lives in a sea of bacteria. Infectious agents known as microbes swim daily throughout our bodies. Microbes can reside in our throat, mouth, gums, nose, gastrointestinal tract, etc. These microorganisms (i.e., bacteria, viruses, fungi) are as much a part of every human being as foods and chemicals. Figuratively speaking, they are constantly trying to "eat us alive." Sometimes they succeed! Even if we die of causes other than infection, they eventually eat our physical remains. Only healthy cells, tissues and organs within our bodies can effectively defend against infectious microorganisms.

Microbes, whether they are bacteria, viruses or fungi, do not usually cause illness until an individual's host resistance declines. "Host resistance" is a technical term used by physicians to describe the complicated mechanisms by which our bodies fight off infections. One of the most important defense mechanisms is the destruction of invading microorganisms by blood leukocytes (white blood cells). These special cells actually ingest microbes and render them harmless. But before leukocytes can be manufactured in the body, there must be an optimum supply of amino acids, vitamins A, C, B1, B2, B6, B12, biotin, niacinamide, pantothenic acid and others, as well as a complete balance of all the minerals and trace elements. If even a single amino acid is deficient or missing, leukocyte production is diminished or may even cease. When this occurs, host resistance within the body is weakened, and a greater susceptibility to infections of all kinds ensues.

Another "host resistance" defense mechanism is the antibody system. When our bodies are receiving optimal nutritional support, specialized protein substances known as antibodies are produced. These substances are constructed from chains of amino acids (protein). Antibodies also attack invading microorganisms and render them susceptible to destruction by the leukocytes. An individual infectious microbe always provokes antibodies that are specifically targeted against that particular type of microbe and no other. Once the body has synthesized specific antibodies, the lymph cells can then reproduce them any time they are needed, provided there are optimum levels of amino acids, vitamins, minerals, trace elements and enzymes from which they can be constructed. Accordingly, if your antibodies for measles, for example, have been synthesized, you will more than likely remain free of measles upon re-exposure to the measles virus. In such a case, your "host resistance" (i.e., a healthy immune system or adequate production of antibodies, leukocytes and phagocytes), maintained via optimum nutritional support, is functioning properly.

It is essential to understand, therefore, that in the real world, infectious illness occurs not because some "germ" arbitrarily decides to attack our bodies. Rather, illness occurs because our nutritionally deficient, debilitated bodies permit these microbes to set up residence. In short, an opportunist microbe is an infectious agent that produces disease only when the circumstances are favorable.

Nutrient deficits can severely impair the integrity of a healthy immune system. Other factors, however, are also critically involved in resistance to infection. The ingestion of large amounts of sugar, for example, paralyzes the phagocytic capacity of our white blood cells. Likewise, when you fail to obtain your needed quota of sleep, resistance to infectious invasion decreases. Similarly, a personal loss, chronic constipation or diarrhea, irritative chemical exposures to the respiratory epithelium, anxiety, too much physical stress, chronic food-chemical allergies and other factors can all influence your resistance to infections. Yet underlying all of these possible causes of poor health are specific nutrient deficiencies which must be individually tested and diagnosed, and then treated according to empirical laboratory findings.

Traditional medical treatment for bacterial infectious flare-up is the administration of antibiotics. Usually little or no advice is given to the patient concerning nutritional support for weakened resistance. And although traditional treatment generally involves drugs that allay symptomatic disorders, the use of drugs does not cure the underlying nutritional-metabolic deficiencies which are usually the fundamental cause of the illness in the first place. To be sure, this is not to argue against the use of antibiotics. At times, they are very helpful and necessary. However, if the nutritional root causes of infectious disease are not treated, illness after illness may continue to occur, and often become worse, as time goes on.

To make matters more disquieting, typical antibiotic medical treatment aimed at the symptomatic relief of infectious flare-up does in fact sometimes produce serious side effects in the form of fungal disorders. The microorganism Candida albicans is one prevalent example of an infectious overgrowth resulting from the repetitive use, or misuse, of antibiotics. We are all indebted to C. Orian Truss, M.D., for alerting us to the frequency, scope and severity of Candida albicans infection. His observations, elaborated in his book *The Missing Diagnosis* (Birmingham, Alabama: C. Orian Truss, M.D., 1983), serve as the basis for the current interest in the detection and treatment of this condition. Another highly recommended book is *The Yeast Connection* by William G. Crook, M.D. (Jackson, Tennessee: Professional Books, 1983).

In its current incarnation, Candida seems to strike women more often than men. Because of the warm, moist conditions in the vagina, that is the area most commonly affected. As is the case with all other forms of infection, a compromised host resistance is the primary cause of Candida albicans. The problem occurs when there is an abnormal fungus yeast growth that is normally controlled by "friendly bacteria" in the intestines. When factors such as antibiotics, steroids (like cortisone), birth control pills and refined sugar are used in excess, "friendly bacteria" and/or specific nutrients in the blood are destroyed. Host resistance is then lowered and the yeast fungi begin to invade and colonize the body's cells, tissues and—finally—organs. A strong, healthy immune system will, of course, contain Candida's growth. Only when host resistance is lowered can Candida invade and colonize the tissues. When colonized, these yeast fungi release toxic chemicals into the blood and cause such varying symptoms as yeast vaginitis, rectal itching, chronic diarrhea or constipation, menstrual cramps and irregularities, bladder infections, lethargy, headaches, acne, severe depression, anxiety, nervousness, mental confusion and others. Toxic chemicals produced by the Candida fungi attack the immune system, permitting the fungi to continue their tissue invasion and to cause more serious symptomatic disorders.

The first Candida infections are usually mild in nature and brief in duration. They may even clear up spontaneously, for when the healthy immune system asserts itself the body returns to normal. In some people, however, the infections recur with increasing frequency. They flourish in the digestive tract, giving rise to colitis and/or esophagitis. Gradually these symptoms, or others, become chronic. The immune system has been challenged so often that it loses its ability to eradicate Candida. Now the body must live with the continued destructive presence of this fungus.

DIAGNOSIS

In order to confirm the presence of candidiasis, one must have a high index of suspicion for the condition. Recognition of the risk factors that predispose one to Candida overgrowth is helpful. These are:

1. pregnancy or multiple pregnancies
2. history of taking birth control pills
3. diabetes mellitus
4. history of taking cortisone (corticosteroids)
5. history of taking antibiotics, especially those of the tetracycline type
6. chemotherapy, irradiation, prolonged illness, debilitation, malnutrition, indwelling catheters, hyperalimentation
7. diet high in sweets, fruits and juices

In addition, the presence of multiple food allergies and chemical sensitivities suggests that candidiasis may well be operative.

Some physicians believe that cultures are not useful in the diagnosis of the Candida albicans syndrome, because they feel that since the organism is ubiquitous, demonstrating its presence is not helpful. The clinical experience of a number of bioecologic physicians suggests otherwise. These physicians take cultures for fungus from the nose, throat, mouth, gums, tongue, anus, rectum, male genitalia, vulva, vagina, groin, armpits, under breasts, and from any skin lesions. Cultures taken repeatedly from a wide variety of patients have shown that the absence of Candida is circumstantial evidence against the Candida albicans syndrome. When the organism is recovered on culture, however, the likelihood that the condition exists is heightened. Furthermore, recovery of a large number of Candida organisms increases the likelihood that the yeast is causing mischief. When cultures are properly taken to avoid contamination, the presence of Candida in the sputum, urine, spinal fluid or blood indicates a serious fungal infection.

Cultures require several days or longer to grow and are therefore not helpful on the day of the test. Another helpful diagnostic tool is a blood test for Candida precipitins (antibodies) by double immunodiffusion. When Candida precipitins are detected, it is evidence for the continued presence of the organism in the patient's body (active infection). Under suitable treatment, the Candida precipitins revert to negative.

Virtually any biological material can be examined under a microscope for detection of fungi. The KOH Prep is another diagnostic tool that may be used on clinical specimens submitted to the laboratory. With this test, an immediate answer can be given as to whether any fungal elements are present or not. A 10 percent solution of potassium hydroxide (KOH) clears debris so that fungal elements can be more readily detected in the specimen. Gently heating the microscopic mount accelerates the process.

Clinical specimens (pus, stool, sputum, vaginal secretions, etc.) can also be smeared and stained on a glass slide. These specimens can be examined on the same day as the sample and the presence or absence of fungal elements can be noted and reported.

At the present stage in our diagnostic capabilities, we may not be able to make a definite diagnosis of candidiasis without a trial of therapy. Accordingly, when the physician's judgment so indicates, a bout of treatment may be needed to confirm diagnostic suspicions. Commonly, a trial of medication is given and the results are carefully monitored.

Candidiasis is the medical term used to describe the yeast fungus overgrowth. It is by no means a new medical problem; in fact, it has been around for centuries. However, candidiasis has become a chronic modern medical dilemma that seems to be increasing rapidly. The reasons for this are the declining vitality of many persons because of several generations of suboptimal diets and the associated factors of drug and chemical exposures.

TREATMENT

Treatment of candidiasis can involve four major steps: First, the yeast fungi must be killed. Second, all immuno-suppressive drugs and antibiotics must be eliminated if possible or used only when absolutely necessary. Third, the diet can be altered to deprive the yeast of food upon which it flourishes. Fourth, and most important of all, the body's weakened nutritionally-based immune system must be strengthened and thus restored to its proper function.

The first part of candidiasis treatment involves the inactivation of the yeast fungi. Nystatin is a very specific drug that kills Candida. It can be used orally, topically, or in the vagina. In most cases, nystatin has been demon-strated to be a safe symptomatic treatment. The following case history, however, reveals that for some people nystatin therapy can be toxic.

A twenty-eight-year-old woman had repeated throat infections and repeated pelvic infections over the course of five years. She was identified by her gynecologist as having pelvic inflammatory disease. She took antibiotics for two to four weeks approximately every two months over a five-year period. Because there was an identified overgrowth of Candida albicans fungus in the vagina of this patient, she was placed on oral nystatin powder and intravaginal nystatin tablets for a one-year period. During this time she had insomnia, felt depressed, anxious, and at times paranoid. When the dose of nystatin was increased, these symptoms became more severe. Conversely, when the dose was decreased, she felt much better. Therefore, after rectal, vaginal and mouth cultures for Candida were found to be negative, nystatin was discontinued. The patient was treated with nutrient supplements, a rotated diet and anti-allergic therapy. Within six months she was more than 75 percent improved, and within a year, she was completely well.

An important caution must be given for patients who are treated with nystatin. At times, the sudden killing of Candida organisms may produce a worsening of symptoms. When this occurs, it tends to confirm the presence of candidiasis but the heightened symptoms may be quite distressing. Alteration in dosage may help. In some cases, alternative treatments must be employed.

Because each case history is different, treatment must be tailored to fit each person's unique situation. Not everyone can tolerate nystatin. It is also important to remember that if only nystatin is used to treat candidiasis, the root causes of the disorder are being ignored and future fungus flare-ups are well within the realm of possibility. In short, nystatin therapy should be viewed as an important but partial and symptomatic treatment of an infectious disorder that requires a complete professionally-monitored nutritional evaluation and follow-up treatment.

Other forms of treatment are available for those who either cannot tolerate nystatin or wish not to take the drug. Ketoconazole (Nizoral, Janssen Pharmaceutica, Inc., New Brunswick, New Jersey) is a broad-spectrum antifungal drug. Although quite effective against Candida when used in adequate dosage, ketoconazole can cause serious liver damage. Other drugs are available for use in very serious cases; however, they may have dangerous side effects and close medical supervision is mandatory.

Many persons today wish to utilize the most natural methods that they can to combat health problems. Fortunately, in the case of Candida vaginitis, there are methods of natural treatment that often work. The woman can douche twice a day with the following mixture: one pint of water to which is added 4 aqueous chlorophyll capsules (available from Standard Process Laboratories, Milwaukee, Wisconsin) and 1 tablespoon of vinegar. At bedtime, insert 2 Zymex wafers (also available from Standard Process Laboratories) in the vagina and wear a pad to keep them in place. Zymex wafers are said to contain a strain of yeast known as lactic acid yeast that inhibits Candida. Lactobacillus acidophilus organisms can also be inserted in the vagina to counter Candida. Care must be taken that potent live cultures of Lactobacilli are used. Intravaginal use of herbs can also effectively combat vaginal Candida infection. One such herbal powder (called V-X) consists of a mixture of squaw vine, chickweed, slippery elm, comfrey, yellow dock, golden seal, mullein and marshmallow (Nature's Sunshine Products, Division of Amtec Industries, Spanish Fork, Utah). These treatments must, of course, be undertaken only with permission and supervision of a physician.

Garlic is also used in treating candidiasis. Researchers at the University of Massachusetts have reported that garlic is highly successful in killing Candida. Since onions are of the same food family as garlic, they may also have the same antifungal properties. Garlic may be taken fresh or in odorless form (e.g., Kyolic, Waukanaga of America Co., Ltd., Honolulu, Hawaii; Garlic Capsules, Miller Pharmaceutical Group, Inc., West Chicago, Illinois). Olive oil and the B vitamin biotin also supress Candida.

While the patient is taking nystatin, ketoconazole, garlic, or one of the other treatment agents, he or she must also avoid immunosuppressive drugs. These include cortisone (corticosteroids) and all forms of oral contraceptives. Moreover, antibiotics, which promote the growth of Candida, must either be eliminated or used only when absolutely necessary.

The power of antibiotics as a tool for fighting bacterial infection is undeniable. Unfortunately, however, they also activate the growth of Candida infection, which is dramatically illustrated by the following case history. A twenty-eight-year-old woman sustained repeated bouts of pelvic infection. For each bout of infection in the tubes and ovaries, antibiotics were administered. After several years of infections and antibiotics, the woman developed itching of the vulva and vagina and a thick white discharge. Cultures of her vagina were positive for Candida albicans. Treatment with nystatin intravaginally resulted in the disappearance of the vaginal discharge and itching. Whenever the nystatin was stopped, the symptoms of yeast vaginitis returned, only to remit again when nystatin treatment was restarted.

Finally, the patient was instructed to continue the nystatin vaginal treatment indefinitely. After one year of treatment the woman was ostensibly well. Vaginal cultures were taken and no fungus was recovered. The nystatin was discontinued and the patient remained free of vaginal symptoms for approximately six months. At that time the woman developed a sore throat with swollen lymph glands. Tetracycline antibiotic was administered for this infection. Within two days, symptoms of vulval and vaginal itching appeared and became severe. Within another few days, thick white vaginal discharge was noted and a culture of the vagina was positive for Candida albicans. Withdrawal of the antibiotic and the administration of intravaginal nystatin suppositories promptly alleviated the vaginal symptoms.

How do antibiotics promote the overgrowth of Candida albicans? They do so by killing off the normal flora indigenous to the gut or the vagina. When these "friendly bacteria" are eradicated, the remaining fungi are left unchecked to proliferate. Evidence for this explanation is provided by the observation that the provision of "friendly bacteria" can counter Candida infection and restore desirable bacterial-fungal balance in some cases. Dr. Truss has also pointed out that Candida eats tetracycline antibiotic, that is, that the yeast can thrive on the antibiotic as a food source (C. Orian Truss, M. D., Yeast-Human Interaction Conference, Birmingham, Alabama, December 9–11, 1983).

Whenever a tetracycline antibiotic is indicated for the treatment of infection, tetracycline combined with the antifungal drug amphotericin B is available (Mysteclin F, E.R. Squibb and Sons, Inc., Princeton, New Jersey). The physician may elect to use this product in order to minimize or prevent fungal overgrowth.

But the avoidance of certain drugs is only a partial answer to complete recovery. A major tool for suppression and eradication of Candida is diet. Candida yeasts thrive when their host eats a diet high in sugars. Thus those persons who consume refined white sugar and honey, and foods that contain them, are inadvertently helping Candida to prosper. Moreover, fruits and fruit juices also provide sugars that serve as food for the unwanted yeast organisms. Dr. Melvin Page, a dentist who pioneered in nutritional research, advocated the virtual elimination of fruits in the diet in order to foster health. His dietary advice is right on the mark for those struggling to inhibit Candida growth.

Some physicians advise the use of a low-carbohydrate diet as a tool of anti-Candida treatment. As low as 60 grams per day has been suggested. Such a diet restricts complex carbohydrates (beans, grains, peas, potatoes, sweet potatoes, some squashes, etc.) as well as fruits. Although this could be helpful, it is commonly unnecessary and indeed may be responsible for worsening an already serious malnutritive condition. In our zeal to help the patient with yeast infection, we must be quite alert to the importance of optimum nutrition. True, we may be able to starve the yeast by one or more particular diets.

However, if we starve the patient at the same time, we are not helping him or her to mount an effective immune defense.

Another dietary alteration that can assist in combating Candida is the prohibition of all foods that contain yeast. Such foods include cheeses, risen bread, sour cream, buttermilk, beer, wine, cider, mushrooms, soy sauce, tofu, vinegar, dried fruits, melons and frozen or canned juices. Some persons may require extensive food avoidances along this line but most do not unless they are specifically known to be yeast-allergic. It should be noted that fruits and fruit juices are also foods that contain yeast organisms. B-complex vitamins are commonly derived from yeast unless specifically noted otherwise.

The prohibition of yeast-containing foods is usually helpful in the clinical management of Candida infections. However, in the authors' experience, yeast-containing foods can sometimes be allowed. Yeast is a very nutritious substance, and certainly, for many persons, the availability of yeast and yeast-containing foods can be a dietary plus that may enable them to avoid non-nutritious sucrose in its more artificial forms. In short, when treating candidiasis, the blanket prohibition of yeast and all yeast-containing foods may not be necessary. Certainly, however, for yeast-sensitive individuals, such a diet is an extremely important clinical tool which must be judiciously implemented.

BUILDING A BETTER DIET

The most important aspect of Candida treatment is repairing the patient's debilitated and nutritionally deficient immune system. This is accomplished by following an individually tailored diet and supplement program, both of which should be tested and monitored by an experienced bioecologic physician.

Bioecologic medicine aims primarily at the achievement and preservation of optimum health and prevention and treatment of infectious as well as degenerative disease by regulating the concentrations of chemical substances normally found in the human body. These substances include minerals, trace elements, vitamins, essential fatty acids, enzymes, amino acids and hormones. This concept implies that the nutritional microenvironment of every one of our body's sixty trillion cells is extremely important to our optimum health, and that deficiencies in this environment constitute the major cause of disease. If deficiencies in the cell develop, as they certainly do with any disease, Candida or otherwise, the theory is that the concentration of these normally occurring chemicals needed for optimum health must be altered in accordance with individual needs. If your body cells are ailing, as they certainly must be in any form of infectious or degenerative disease, chances are excellent that it is because they are not being adequately provided with the optimum nutrients, enzymes or hormones they need to sustain and propagate healthy tissues, organs and life in general. Infections that demand antibiotic treatment do not arise *de novo* out of the air. Most of the time infections occur because host immunity is poor. And most of the time this occurs because of faulty diet and nutrient deficiencies.

As already explained, dietary measures that have been advocated for candidiasis include the avoidance of sweet foods as well as the elimination of foods that contain yeast. Certainly it does seem desirable to practice a reasonable degree of dietary abstinence from sweets. For we do not believe it to be coincidental that we have an extremely high nationwide consumption of refined sugar and a virtual epidemic of Candida and related yeast infections. (See Ray C. Wunderlich, Jr., M.D., *Sugar and Your Health* [St. Petersburg, Fla.: Johnny Reads, Inc., 1982], p. 21.) The term "sweets," of course, includes all the refined sugar-containing foods such as candies, cakes, ice cream, many soft drinks, catsup and Jello. On the other hand, if the diet contains ample quantities of fresh whole foods (for example, seeds, nuts, vegetables and whole grains), then the sugar-laden foods should be minimal, and the chances of developing Candida albicans infection will be considerably reduced.

Certain dietary guidelines can be put forth that will promote health when they are faithfully followed. These guidelines are as follows:

1. Eat fresh whole foods.
2. Eat a wide variety of foods in a diversified pattern.
3. Eat no foods that are toxic, allergic or metabolically offensive.
4. Eat neither too much nor too little food.

No person can eat perfectly. Nevertheless, these guidelines serve as a sturdy scaffold for the individual who wishes to climb higher toward the nutritional optimum.

Other factors which definitely help to build the immune system are nutritional supplements. For the candidiasis patient, preparations free of sugar, cornstarch, dyes and yeast must be used. Nutrients that are known to support the immune system are, to mention a few, vitamins C, E, A, B6 and pantothenic acid, as well as zinc, selenium, specific amino acids and essential fatty acids. It is not within the scope of this brief manual to cover each of these nutrients in depth. It is important to understand, however, that before anyone begins taking any vitamin, mineral or amino acid, he or she should be individually evaluated by a knowledgeable professional for specific deficiencies. Each human being's nutritional needs are distinctive and appreciably different from those of others. Just because specific nutrients helped one individual's resistance to infectious disease does not necessarily guarantee another person's increased resistance to disease if he follows the same program.

Additionally, it is sometimes dangerous to take only one or two specific nutrients while disregarding all the others. Nutrients, in contrast to drugs, work together as a team in building health and optimum resistance to infectious disease. Accordingly, the physiological effects of drugs can be ascribed to their singular ability to enter into metabolic machinery and interfere with specific enzyme systems. Nutrients, on the other hand, act constructively as building blocks for all enzyme systems. Therefore, nutrients as physiological agents must be judged on the basis of how effectively they build health as team players. In each individual case history, prescribed amounts of vitamins, minerals, trace elements, amino acids and hormones must be tailored according to specific needs and then given in a balanced formula. An experienced bio-ecologic physician is best qualified to do this. For a more detailed account of this important topic, see chapter 9 of *Nourishing Your Child* by the present authors (New Canaan, Connecticut: Keats Publishing, Inc., 1984).

Sometimes the physician utilizes immunotherapy to build a capable immune defense against yeast. Extracts of Candida as well as other fungi can be injected into the patient to build immunity. For some persons, immunotherapy can be most helpful, but it is usually an adjunct and may not be needed when nutritional measures are properly invoked.

The herb Taheebo is an example of a remedy that boosts immune defenses and is sometimes effective in the treatment of candidiasis as well as other infections. Taheebo tea (it is sometimes called La Pacho or Pau D'Arco) is a flavorful tea made from the inner bark of a Brazilian plant. Some believe its efficacy is due to direct antifungal action. However, it is more likely that Taheebo's anti infectious action derives from stimulation of the host's imm̄ne system in an as yet unknown manner.

After drinking Taheebo tea, Gail F. Nielson reported in *The Human Ecologist* (North Bend, Washington: The Communicate Company, 1983, p. 4) that she was able to stop taking her previously required nystatin without experiencing any Candida-related symptomatology:

> I began fourteen months ago to drink Taheebo tea. After experiencing a marked improvement over the next four months . . . I have been completely off nystatin for seven months. I am now leading a "normal life"! Some Candida sufferers have reported some pleasant side effects from drinking Taheebo tea. One man's chronic athlete's foot cleared up within one month, while another experienced the clearing of skin rashes on his head, face and hands. Still another patient's fungus-ridden nails cleared after two months of Taheebo tea treatment.

Taheebo tea acts as a diuretic, and the patient who continues to drink it for a period of time may wish to supplement his diet with additional sodium, calcium, potassium and magnesium as well as other minerals and trace elements. Obviously, professional monitoring of body mineral levels is advised.

Case history 1: Vaginitis

A fifty-three-year-old housewife had a fifteen-year history of recurrent vaginal yeast infections. She was treated each time by her gynecologist with intravaginal nystatin. Each time she was treated, her symptoms of severe vaginal itching, pain and discharge promptly disappeared. A program of enhanced local hygiene was instituted and daily Lactobacillus acidophilus douching was prescribed. The patient was placed on a special diet and given appropriate supplements. No further vaginal yeast infections occurred. The additional nutritional support increased her resistance to Candida, and thus eliminated the continual reappearance of the yeast infection.

A number of factors may be responsible for precipitating Candida vaginal infection. Warmth, wetness, improper hygiene, improper nutrition, low immune-system response, birth control pills, antibiotics and cortisone (corticosteroids) can all contribute to this infectious disease. Those who live in the southern part of the United States are more likely to encounter significant fungus infections than their counterparts in the north, probably because of the warmth and humidity so common in the southern states. (In Florida, for example, from April to October, there is a marked increase in the numbers of symptomatic vaginal infections due to Candida.) Outer as well as underclothing should be chosen so that excessive sweating is avoided as much as possible, particularly in the perineal area (the region between the thighs at the outlet of the pelvis).

Candida vaginitis can be a venereal disease, since it can be transmitted from partner to partner by sexual activity. The male may harbor Candida on or around his genitals and introduce the fungus into the female at the time of sexual intercourse. Likewise, the male may contract Candida from an infected partner. Some cases of chronic or recurrent Candida vaginitis occur because the infected sexual partner has not been treated.

Perfumes used in the name of feminine hygiene, as well as dyes in toilet papers, may cause vulval irritation, which may, in turn, act as a nonspecific inciter of vulvovaginal candidiasis. Allergic vaginitis is not a rare condition and may underlie Candida infection.

As mentioned previously, the use of antibiotics may cause candidiasis. Any antibiotic worth its salt will eradicate Lactobacillus organisms in the gastrointestinal tract and in the vagina also. A woman's vagina cannot maintain a healthy state without the presence of Lactobacillus acidophilus organisms. During birth, in fact, the mother's vagina, which hosts Lactobacilli, introduces these "friendly bacteria" into the baby's gut to protect the infant from pathogenic bacteria. Antibiotic-altered flora in the gut and/or vagina must therefore be considered a major precipitant of vaginal Candida infection.

Incorrect wiping after using the toilet is the number one method of spreading fungi from the gastrointestinal tract to the female genitalia. Many women wipe from the back to the front, that is, from the anus toward the vulva. This practically ensures that any Candida resident in the bowel can gain access to the warm, moist, recessed female genital tract. The opposite direction of wiping is obviously the preferred method.

Candida infections commonly commence in the ten-to fourteen-day interval following ovulation and flare up in the days immediately following a menstrual period. The female hormone progesterone, a component of birth control pills, enhances Candida growth. It is in relative excess in the postovulatory days. The postmenstrual flare is not surprising since blood is an excellent culture medium. The use of tampons may also be a fungus activator. A tampon is a foreign body used in a warm cavity filled with stale blood.

What can we recommend for the woman who wishes to do everything possible to preserve host integrity and prevent Candida infection? First, she can see to it that her body contains Lactobacillus organisms. This is done preferably, of course, by not eradicating them in the first place with antibiotics. (An improved lifestyle with strict adherence to the four dietary guidelines given in this text will eliminate the need for most antibiotics.) Lactobacillus acidophilus may be taken orally as a dietary supplement. Implants of Lactobacilli can also be placed in the vagina and/or colon. Second, women can wear skirts to permit air circulation. Cotton underclothes will be cool as well as absorbent. Third, meticulous hygiene helps to avoid vaginal contamination with Candida. This includes wiping after toilet from the front to the back, frequent changes of tampons or pads (every few hours) during menses, and frequent bathing. Fourth, vinegar douches (1 tablespoon vinegar to 1 quart of water) may help to acidify the vagina, but the effects are short-lived. The use of Acigel (Ortho Pharmaceutical Corporation, Raritan, New Jersey) at bedtime, under professional supervision, is, however, quite effective. With appropriate vaginal acidification, Candida albicans is less likely to become bothersome. Fifth, women should empty their bladders before having sexual intercourse. Avoidance of oral-genital sex is also advised. After sexual relations, the woman should cleanse her perineal area. And finally, the overgrowth of Candida albicans is also related to the pH of the body. The pH of the vagina in the normal adult woman is distinctly acid (i.e., from 4 to 5). The vagina becomes alkaline during menstruation, since the pH of blood is 7.4. Vaginal pH in the presence of infections is also alkaline or relatively alkaline. Vaginal infection due to Candida albicans is no exception. Thus, the presence of an alkaline pH in the vagina of the nonmenstruating woman can be considered circumstantial evidence for the presence of Candida. Vaginal pH should be monitored by a professional.

Case history 2: Sore tongue

A sixty-two-year-old woman had complained of a sore tongue for ten years. Many vitamin treatments had been taken through the years but resulted in little or no improvement. The woman had consulted a number of physicians, dentists and naturopaths and had religiously followed their advice, but to no avail. She complained of a constantly burning tongue and a feeling of fullness in the tongue. The last physician she consulted had administered a course of injectable vitamins, but there was no improvement.

Examination of the tongue showed swelling and redness, and deep furrows with a white coating. The gums were also swollen and red. Scrapings of the tongue's surface, suspended in potassium hydroxide and examined under a microscope, showed fragments typical of fungus. Cultures of the gums, tongue, throat, rectum and vagina were positive for Candida albicans. Antibodies (precipitins) for Candida were detected in the blood. A prick test of the skin for Candida albicans was strongly positive.

Treatment against Candida fungus was started with powdered nystatin taken by mouth. Within one week the woman reported the disappearance of the burning sensation in her tongue. Coincidentally, she reported that her digestion had improved and she was sleeping better at night. According to her husband, her disposition had also improved.

Repeat laboratory tests taken after two months of continued treatment disclosed negative cultures for fungus and an absence of Candida antibodies in the blood. At the present time, the woman's body chemistry and immune system are being strengthened by nutritional means.

Case history 3: Infant colic

Robert was challenging for his parents because of his chronic irritability. Awake at night, troubled with gas and cramps during the day, this nine-week-old infant also spit up his milk and frequently had diarrhea. Multiple changes of formula were tried to alleviate his gastrointestinal problems and irritability, but there was no discernible improvement. The mother was advised to give the infant anticolic drops that contained phenobarbital and belladonna. This medication calmed the infant but after each dose wore off, he was even more troubled with cramps and gas than he was when the drops were not given.

The mother reported to the child's physician that she herself was continuously troubled with recurrent vaginal fungus infections. Because of this history, the doctor suggested that the infant be given a trial of antifungal medication. A stool culture was taken and reported as positive for the presence of Candida albicans. Nystatin oral drops were started and within two days the infant was noticeably less flatulent and much more comfortable. Within a few weeks, spitting up had disappeared, bowel movements were more regular and less frequent, and he was sleeping comfortably through the night.

Case history 4: Food hypersensitivity

A thirty-six-year-old woman had been ill for ten years since the birth of her only child. She was hypersensitive to many foods and chemicals. Her symptoms included diarrhea, skin eruption, itching, hives, depression, paranoia, dizziness, flatulence, nausea, abdominal bloating, disorientation, low energy and falling hair. She also complained of constant vaginal yeast infections.

Numerous medical investigations had been carried out with negative results. Food eliminations had been performed on numerous occasions. The patient was becoming weaker and more ill with increasing numbers of symptoms associated with food and chemical exposures.

Upon questioning, the woman related that she had been treated with various kinds of antibiotics for acne for many years.

The cluster of food and chemical sensitivities with a history of prolonged antibiotic therapy and recurrent vaginal yeast infections is a classic history for symptom-provoking candidiasis. The onset of the patient's symptoms after pregnancy suggests that Candida overgrowth may have been present since that time. Pregnancy, a high-progesterone state, is a condition that favors Candida growth. Falling hair may be due to malnutrition, toxicity, or hypothyroidism but it is encountered again and again in the histories of patients who have candidiasis.

This woman was given a therapeutic trial of nystatin with full expectation that she would have a good result. Indeed she did. Within a month her assemblage of symptoms was markedly reduced in number and severity. At that time, nutrient supplementation, customized to the patient's needs, was given. Further improvement occurred. A few months later she was able to enlarge her restricted diet. As she became better nourished, her symptoms further abated. She broadened her range of activities as she gained strength. Within a year she was essentially symptom-free.

Which came first in this case? Allergy? Nutrient deficiency? Candida infection? That's like asking which came first, the chicken or the egg. The interaction between yeast organisms and human chemistry is delicately poised. The balance can be upset in many different ways. Commonly, multiple variables coexist to tip the scales in favor of Candida. Once established, Candida in the gut can open up channels in the bowel wall that permit entry of foods into the body and thus bring about allergic response. Also, the Candida organism can suppress the patient's immune system powerfully. Somehow, chemical sensitivities emerge. The patient feels bad, eats poorly, avoids symptom-producing foods and becomes increasingly undernourished. In such a state, conditions are ripe for continued yeast proliferation.

Case history #5: Anal itching

A sixty-year-old man consulted a physician because of intolerable anal itching. Examination showed intense inflammation of the skin around the anus. An anal skin scraping disclosed many fungal fragments and a culture grew Candida albicans.

Additional complaints of difficult swallowing, nausea and heartburn led to a barium X-ray examination of the esophagus. Ragged irregularities were identified consistent with Candida esophagitis. Candida albicans was grown from material hawked up from the man's throat. The man's history revealed that he had been treated with corticosteroid drugs for a considerable period of time because of a severe asthmatic condition. He was also known to have diabetes mellitus.

Treatment with nystatin was undertaken but did not help. Ketoconazole along with the institution of a program of nutrient management relieved his symptoms. Also, his asthma improved to the extent that corticosteroid drugs were not required.

Candida had overgrown in this man from throat to anus. Corticosteroids, diabetes, and nutrient inadequacies teamed to promote the fungal proliferation. Successful treatment suggested that candidiasis may have been a factor in worsening the asthma.

A high index of suspicion on the part of the patient and the physician will help to counter Candida albicans, the opportunistic pathogen that waits in the wings to cause distress.

CONCLUSION

In summary, Candida albicans is a yeast fungus that takes advantage of circumstances in a person's body that are conducive to its growth. It becomes disease-producing when host resistance is compromised. The most important factors leading to a susceptibility of this particular kind are: use and overuse of antibiotics, birth control pills or cortisone (corticosteroids); pregnancy and multiple pregnancies; diabetes mellitus; nutritive deficiencies and other debilitated states; and a lack of meticulous hygiene. When optimal nourishment and meticulous hygiene are employed, we should be able to reduce drastically the need for antibiotics, corticosteroids and antifungal medication.

Many encouraging signs indicate that at long last a renaissance of nutritional science is imminent: Thousands of physicians, medical students and laymen are becoming very interested in studying the field of nutrition and its relation to human disease. Bioecologic physicians believe that through the proper use of optimum nutrition, our host resistance can be improved to the point at which our normal healthy bodily processes can indeed fight off infections of all kinds, including Candida albicans.

62 Inexpensive Booklets to Build a Full-Spectrum Health Library

GOOD HEALTH GUIDES

Aloe Vera, Jojoba and Yucca
John Heinerman — **$1.95**

The Antioxidants
Richard A. Passwater, Ph.D. — **$1.95**

Ask Jeanne Rose About Herbs
Jeanne Rose — **$1.45**

The Bach Remedies A Self-Help Guide
Leslie J. Kaslof — **$1.95**

A Beginner's Introduction to Homeopathy
Trevor M. Cook, Ph.D. — **$1.95**

A Beginner's Introduction to Nutrition
Albrecht A. Heyer — **$1.95**

A Beginner's Introduction to Trace Minerals
Erwin DiCyan, Ph.D. — **$1.95**

A Beginner's Introduction to Vitamins
Richard A. Passwater, Ph.D. — **$1.95**

Beta-Carotene
Richard A. Passwater, Ph.D. — **$1.95**

Bioflavonoids
Jeffrey Bland, Ph.D. — **$1.95**

Brewer's Yeast, Wheat Germ and Other High Power Foods
Beatrice Trum Hunter — **$1.95**

Candida Albicans
Ray C. Wunderlich Jr., M.D. and Dwight K. Kalita, Ph.D. — **$1.95**

Chlorella
William H. Lee, R.Ph., Ph.D. and M. Rosenbaum, M.D. — **$1.95**

Choline, Lecithin, Inositol and Other "Accessory" Nutrients (Vol. 1)
Jeffrey Bland, Ph.D. — **$1.95**

Coenzyme Q-10
William H. Lee, R.Ph., Ph.D. — **$1.95**

Dietary Fiber
Shirley S. Lorenzani, Ph.D. — **$1.95**

Digestive Enzymes
Jeffrey Bland, Ph.D. — **$1.95**

The Disease of Aging
Hans Kugler, Ph.D. — **$1.95**

EPA—Marine Lipids
Richard A. Passwater, Ph.D. — **$1.95**

Esencia de Cebada Verde
Yoshihide Hagiwara, M.D. — **$2.50**

Evening Primrose Oil
Richard A. Passwater, Ph.D. — **$1.95**

First Aid with Herbs
John Heinerman — **$1.95**

Fish Oils Update
Richard A. Passwater, Ph.D. — **$1.95**

The Friendly Bacteria
William H. Lee, R.Ph., Ph.D. — **$1.95**

Gluten Intolerance
Beatrice Trum Hunter — **$1.95**

Green Barley Essence
Yoshihide Hagiwara, M.D. — **$1.95**

GTF Chromium (Glucose Tolerance Factor)
Richard A. Passwater, Ph.D. — **$1.95**

Herbs and Herbal Medicine
William H. Lee, R.Ph., Ph.D. — **$1.95**

How to Cope with Menstrual Problems
Nikki Goldbeck — **$1.95**

Hypoglycemia
Marilyn Light — **$1.95**

Kelp, Dulse and Other Sea Supplements
William H. Lee, R.Ph., Ph.D. — **$1.95**

Lifetime Wellness
Joan A. Friedrich, Ph.D. — **$1.95**

Lysine, Tryptophan and Other Amino Acids
Robert Garrison, Jr., R.Ph., M.A. — **$1.95**

The Medicinal Benefits of Mushrooms
William H. Lee, R.Ph., Ph.D., Teruaki Hayashi, Ph.D. and Yasuo Hotta, D.Sc. — **$1.95**

Nutrition and Behavior
Alexander Schauss, M.A. — **$1.95**

Nutrition and Exercise for the Over 50s
Susan Smith Jones, Ph.D. — **$1.45**

Nutrition and Stress
Harold Rosenberg, M.D. — **$1.95**

A Nutritional Guide for the Problem Drinker Ruth M. Guenther, Ph.D. — **$1.95**	**Siberian Ginseng** Betty Kamen, Ph.D. — **$1.95**
Nutritional Parenting Sara Sloan — **$1.95**	**Spirulina** Jack Joseph Challem — **$1.95**
Octacosanol, Carnitine and Other "Accessory" Nutrients (Vol. 2) Jeffrey Bland, Ph.D. — **$1.45**	**A Stress Test for Children** Jerome Vogel, M.D. — **$1.45**
Orotates and Other Mineral Transporters William H. Lee, R.Ph., Ph.D. — **$1.95**	**Tofu, Tempeh, Miso and Other Soyfoods** Richard Leviton — **$1.95**
Propolis: Nature's Energizer Carlson Wade — **$1.95**	**Vitamin B3 (Niacin)** Abram Hoffer, M.D, Ph.D. — **$1.45**
The Rinse Formula Jacobus Rinse, Ph.D. — **$1.95**	**Vitamin C Updated** Jack Joseph Challem — **$1.95**
Selenium Update Richard A. Passwater, Ph.D. — **$1.95**	**Vitamin E Updated** Len Mervyn, Ph.D. — **$1.45**
Sesame Betty Kamen, Ph.D. — **$1.95**	**The Vitamin Robbers** Earl Mindell, R.Ph., Ph.D. and H. Lee, R.Ph., Ph.D. — **$1.95**
	Wheat, Millet and Other Grains Beatrice Trum Hunter — **$1.95**

THE SPORTS & FITNESS LIBRARY

Sports Nutrition Walt Evans, M.Ed. — **$2.95**	**Introduction to Body Sculpting** Kevin Lawrence and Diana Dennis with Dr. Bill Lee — **$2.95**
Winning Without Steroids Gayle Olinekova — **$2.95**	**You Can't Lose!** Guy S. Fasciana, M.S., M.Ed. — **$2.95**

THE SELF-CARE HEALTH LIBRARY

Assess Your Own Nutritional Status Jeffrey Bland, Ph.D. — **$2.25**	**Intestinal Toxicity and Inner Cleansing** Jeffrey Bland, Ph.D. — **$2.25**
Evaluate Your Own Biochemical Individuality Jeffrey Bland, Ph.D. — **$2.25**	**Recognize and Manage Your Allergies** Doris J. Rapp, M.D. — **$2.25**

Available from Your Health or Bookstore or from Keats Publishing, Inc.

Write us for a complete catalog
of hardbound and paperback health books.

27 Pine Street (PO Box 876)
New Canaan, CT 06840